I am honored to present

„Your Guide to Positive Life"

It's the first one in a series of workbooks that will help you to change your life, improve your habits and get to know yourself better.

Thanks to our work together, you will:
- Find a positive vibe and wake up every day full of vital energy and joy!
- Discover that it's never too late to make your dreams come true.
- Reduce the level of stress caused by overworking and toxic relationships
- Become calmer and improve your self-confidence.
- Find out which path towards self improvement works best for you.

What if I told you that you can become a person you always wanted to be? How would you feel about it?

All of these are only the small changes that can help you cultivate better habits!
You can find out all by yourself.

Now it's your time. Time to get control on
- your life, your health, your relationships, your dreams!

Remember! You're doing it for yourself.

I wish you all the luck in your journey!
Kasia Dorosz

The order of content:

How to work with *The Guid?* 3
Daily schedule 4
    Morning routine 4
    Evening routine 5
    Weekly assignments 6
1. Gratefulness 7
2. The value of motivational quotes 9
3. Positive attitude 11
4. How to keep the high energy? 13
5. Setting the goals 15
6. Strong will 17
7. Remember – always be yourself! 19
8. Mental resistance 21
9. Motivation as a lifestyle 23
10. Self-esteem 25
11. What is empathy? 27
12. Forgiveness 29
13. Effective motivational techniques 31
14. Stay in touch with yourself 32
15. Don't waste your energy on low self-esteem 35
16. Carpe Diem - enjoy you life! 37

Copyright © 2019 Katarzyna Dorosz

No part of this publication may be reproduced, stored in a retrieval system, or transmitted in any form or by any means, electronic, mechanical, photocopied, recorded, scanned without the prior written permission of the author.

How to work with The Guide

To make the most of the exercises you need:

1. A book with quotes

While working with the Guide, use a book with inspirational quotes, Holy Scriptures, or other reading that you find valuable. I will show you how valuable it is to spend time on contemplating valuable content.

If you need a bit of help on how to feed your spirit to get you started, I encourage you to read my book 101 Sentencji na Każdy Dzień, available in my online store Acti50.tv.

2. A notebook

This workbook includes many questions that answers to which you may want to write down for future reference. It's important to find some time to do it every day. When you write with pen on paper, your brain processes information differently than when you consider it quietly inside your head. This way you will achieve better results in working on your happiness

3. A book calendar/organizer

Write down your conclusions and thoughts at the end of each day. Give yourself time to make it part of your daily routine. At the beginning you can write down all the little goals that you achieved that day. How did you feel while completing them? What sensations did you observe in your body during exercises and contemplation? Maybe one of the thoughts or quotes moved you or maybe you want to write down what you are grateful for today? Every day write down at least one little positive thing that happened to you.

At the end of the week get back to all your notes – you will see how much improvement you've made.
Remember! Your thoughts are worth writing down!

Daily schedule
Below are morning and evening exercises that you can easily introduce into your routine in just one week.

You will start every day full of motivation and vital energy. Your body and mind will liven up. Meanwhile, evenings will be full of fulfilment and gratefulness after a productive day. Your body and mind will relax to get ready for healthy and refreshing sleep.

If you need a little help to stay motivated, write down these exercises on a sticky note place them on the bathroom mirror to help you remember them at all times. When they become your routine – you won't need the reminders anymore.

Morning routine
1. **Practice gratefulness.**
   Feel grateful right after waking up. Finish the following sentence: „I am grateful for..." or just repeat „Thank you" multiple times. Focusing on the good around you will help you begin your the day joyfully.

2. **Read motivational sentences.**
   Read one of your motivational sentences and contemplate its meaning in silence. Focus on the value that it could bring into your life. Feed your heart!

3. **Contemplat.**
   Sit down in a comfortable position. Focus on your breath and heartbeat. Feel your entire body. Stay in silence for 10-20 minutes.
   The beginnings of contemplation may be difficult. Everybody feels that way. Distractions and the sudden flow of thoughts in your head are a normal thing. With time, you will find it easier to focus in silence.
   For motivation and support in furthering your contemplation practice, check out the "Art of Proper Breathing" video, which you can find on the Acti50.tv channel.

4. **Exercises for a good day.**
   You've already fed your heart and mind. It's time to take care of your body. Do some of your favorite physical exercises. Let your body know that a new day has come and you need strength to face it.
   If you're looking for some inspiration - check out the Acti50 YouTube channel.

5. **Affirmations.**
   Affirmations are the positive statements the daily repetitions of which are beneficial to your sense of wellbeing. They boost your self-acceptance by helping you notice the best things about yourself. You can repeat every day: „I am smart!", „I deserve the respect!", „I am a valuable person!", „I deserve the best things!". Add more of your own affirmations.

Evening routine

1. **Relaxing exercises.**
   It's a good time to take care of your body. Do a few relaxing exercises to get rid of the tension and stress that may have occured during the day.

2. **Evening contemplation.**
   Find a comfortable position. Calm down your thoughts. Focus on your breath. Let go of everything that happened during the day.

3. **Filling in your calendar.**
   Write down the good things that happened to you during the day, your thoughts about the exercises you did and the changes you start noticing as a result. Answer the questions: „What am I grateful for today?", „What good did I do today?", „What have I learned today?". Write down one positive thoughts from the day.

4. Gratefulness and good sleep.
  - Close your day with gratitude.
  - If you face difficulties and problems during the day, repeat with me: „God, I am trusting you with my problems. Please, take care of them and give me the right solution in the morning". God will take the best care of your struggles. Leave all your problems behind.

Now, when you are calm, free from the worries, and filled with trust and love for yourself and the world, go to bed. Sleep well.

Weekly assignments

Every week, we will work on four topics. Set a time every day to focus in peace and quiet on the materials I have prepared for you. Work on them conscientiously, following the right sequence of activities.

Week I	Gratefulness	The value of motivational quotes	Positive attitude	How to keep the high energy?
Week II	Setting the goals	Strong will	Remember - always be yourself!	Mental resistance
Week III	Motivation as a lifestyle	Self estcem	What is empathy?	Forgiveness
Week IV	Effective motivational techniques	Staying in touch with yourself	Don't waste your energy on low self esteem?	Carpe diem – enjoy you life!

1. GRATEFULNESS

To start your journey towards happiness you need to realize that it is already there, all around and inside of you.

1. What makes you smile? What is the source of your joy? **Write down three things that make you happy.** It can be a long walk, time spent with a good book, meeting with kind people. Use it to treat yourself as often as possible.

2. **Practice gratefulness.** Finish the sentences:
   I am grateful for...
   I am happy, because...
   I am grateful for this moment, because...

3. **Do you have people around you, who you can be grateful for?** Write down their names in your notebook and then write down what you value in your relationship. Then call them or set up a meeting.

4. **Are you grateful for your body?** Regardless of age, we often find our bodies not good enough and not attractive enough. Accepting your own body is necessary in order to accept yourself, and therefore to find happiness. **Write down three positive thoughts you have about your body.**

   In my case those would be:
   - I am grateful for my skin, because it protects me from the cold and the sun's heat.
   - I am grateful for the way I look, because it makes me unique.
   - I am grateful for my healthy body.

5. Remember about your morning and evening rituals. Write down all the conclusions in your notebook or calendar.

Your Guide to Positive Life

2. THE VALUE OF MOTIVATIONAL QUOTES

Go to the library or a bookstore and get a book with motivational or inspirational quotes. You can also use my „*101 sentences for each day*" which you will find in the Acti50.tv store.

- Sit down in a quiet, comfortable spot.
- Stop for a minute at every quote you read.
- Which of your own life experiences do these quotes apply to?
- Write down the quote that you find the most touching on a small piece of paper and keep it with you at all times.

Examples of quotes you may find worth considering:

1. „*What you are shapes the world in which you live. When you change, the world and the reality around you change as well.*"

2. „*A man's age is the age of their thoughts and feelings.*"

3. „*A man who learns grows younger and one who stops learning grows older.*"

4. „*If you want something you have not had in your life yet, you have to do something that you have never done yet.*" - Thomas Jefferson

5. „*Your life gets better only when you become better!*" - Brian Tracy

6. „*The main skill in life is to find the golden mean. It's about the balance between our plans and what happens to us in real life. It is important to make the right choices and decisions and to respond appropriately to the facts and events that happen to us. Focus on the optimal use of every moment you have.*"

7. „*Weigh carefully your thoughts and the words you say. Think only positive thoughts, because your subconscious does not have a sense of humour and makes true every thing that you believe.*"

Your Guide to Positive Life

3. POSITIVE ATTITUDE

JPositive attitude is necessary if you really want to change your life. It will give you the strenght to face problems. It's time to focus more carefully on everyday affirmations and good thoughts about yourself.

Make your own list and always keep it with you, use it whenever you need support. Affirmations create our reality, so after some time you won't need them anymore. Positive thinking will become your natural habit.

Take a look at my list – if you want it, you can use it as inspiration:

- Every day I feel joy and strength to face life.
- I enjoy my work, everyday tasks and responsibilities.
- I am a wise and valuable person.
- I manage my time wisely.
- I have a lot of vital energy!
- I am fully focused on and engaged in the thing I am doing at the moment. I enjoy doing it.
- I always find some time for myself.
- I love other people, and they love me back.
- I take care of my health every day.
- I feel young every day.

Your Guide to Positive Life

4. WAYS TO KEEP HIGH LEVELS OF ENERGY

This is a question you ask me a lot and I will talk about it more in the second part of the Guide. Meanwhile open your notebook and make a table:

I feel energized when:	I lose my energy when:

Write down every answer that comes to your mind!
Now you know, how to save your energy! Make sure that as many things as possible give you energy during the day - you already have a whole list. At the same time, one by one eliminate from your life the things that take it away from you.

I have a few suggestions more:

1. Start your day with a happy shout out: „It's going to be a great day!".
2. Practice affirmations – you already know how to do it.
3. During the day, find time for a quiet moment.
   You can do it by reducing the amount of time you spend watching TV and using the computer. Remember to use your phone only to talk, not to browse social media.
4. Think positively.
5. Learn to set goals.
   We are going to work on this together.
6. Spend time with valuable people.
7. When you experience a drop in energy, do something stimulating – a cold shower works best for me, I guarantee immediate improvement!

Your Guide to Positive Life

5. SETTING THE GOALS

If you have had a problem achieving your goals, then the following tips will definitely help you.

Four tips for setting te goals

1. **Divide a big goal into several smaller ones.**
   If you are using this Guide, you certainly have at least one goal – a healthy and happy life. It is very ambitious, so together we will divide it into smaller steps: first, we will introduce gratefulness and positive thinking. Thanks to this, you will have enough strength and enthusiasm to continue working on yourself. Right now, you are learning to set goals and achieve them. Taking notes in your calendar helps you notice your progress. This leaves no room for discouragement!

2. **Reward yourself.**
   Positive feedback in itself is a reward. Share your achievements with people who care about you. You can also send me an email, telling me about what you have achieved. Maybe successfully meditated for the first time? It's worth celebrating!

3. **Change your attitude towards challenges.**
   I will keep encouraging you to take up physical activity. However, if you want to run, but you think you're not strong enough, then go for a walk. Or maybe start with nordic walking? See if there are organized communities in your city. Your body will be grateful. Change your attitude towards challenges!

4. **Use visual reminders.**
   Keep a picture of what you want to achieve in a visible place. You want to start eating healthy? Put a photo of fruit and vegetables on your fridge. Want to be happy every day? Smile and take a selfie to remind you it's possible!

In your notebook, create a plan for your current goal using the steps above.

Your Guide to Positive Life

6. STRONG WILL

Even the best planned goal has no chance to be accomplished without you exercising your willpower. Let's try to analyse why you have had issues with taking care of your health before now.

Consider the following questions and write your truthful answers in a notebook:

1. **What is keeping me from eating healthy? Why it is happening?**
   Maybe you don't have any ideas for tasty snacks or you only associate healthy eating with expensive organic food?

2. **Why can't I keep the proper body weight? What is the REAL cause?**
   Maybe it's the lack of daily exercise or the misleading way of thinking: „I'm too old, I don't have to take care of myself anymore"? Maybe you olny like exercise when you can watch it on TV?

3. **What has my physical activity looked like so far? What are my habits in terms of physical movement?**
   Remember! Physical activity is not just the daily dose of exercise. It's also taking a walk or taking the stairs instead of the elevator.

4. **How do I hydrate my body?**
   Do you drink the right amount of water during the day? Or are you substituting it with coffee?

5. **What does my sleep look like?**
   Think about whether your fatigue is due to the lack of proper routine to wind down before bedtime.

Once you know the underlying causes for your actions, it's going to be easier to find solutions to the problems. Or maybe you can already see the potential to change? Write it down and implement it immediately.

Your Guide to Positive Life

7. REMEMBER - ALWAYS BE YOURSELF!

Although we're working together to make your life better – full of energy and joy – you need to know one thing: - **YOU HAVE VALUE THE WAY YOU ARE.**

You are a diamond that only needs a little polishin. Get rid of everything that makes your life harder and be yourself completely. Today's exercises will help you discover your true self.

1. Read the following sentences and write down which of them appeal to you the most, and why:
   - It all starts with the thought: *"Life consists of what one thinks about throughout the day"* - Ralph Waldo Emerson.

   - What we think determines who we are. Who we are determines what we do: *"People's actions are the best interpreters of their thoughts"* - John Locke.

   - Our thoughts determine our destiny. Our destiny defines our legacy: *"Today, you are wherever your thoughts have taken you. Tomorrow, you will be wherever they cross your mind"* - James Allen.

   - *"Nothing is as embarrassing as watching someone succeed after you said it can not be done"* - Ralph Waldo Emerson.

2. Take time to think about your spiritual life. What are your values? What is the most important thing in your life? Do you follow it every day? Describe your thoughts.

3. Based on the answers to the exercises in Chapter 6, **create a list of things that you would like to improve in yourself.** Do it on a clean sheet and sign it with your name and date when you're done, thus declaring: "Yes, I will strive to be like that!".

Remember about your morning and evening rituals. Always write down the conclusions in your notebook or calendar.

Your Guide to Positive Life

8. MENTAL RESILIENCE

It's worth to focusing on your mental resilience. It's going to help you enjoy good health for a longer period of time, get more satisfaction from your everyday tasks, or have more distance towards yourself and the people around you.

To strengthen your mental resilience, remember:

1. **Commitment is key!**
   The more involved you are in your activities and the goals you want to achieve, the easier it is for you to confront the difficulties.

2. **Create achievable goals.**
   Each completed goal strengthens your psyche. It's a simple message: "It worked! I can achieve whatever I had planned! I have a goal in my life!"

3. **Be assertive.**
   Assertiveness is not only the ability to say „no", it is above all the art of expressing your needs which support your spiritual progress.

4. **Be empathetic.**
   A loving look on yourself and other people makes us stronger.

As you work with your exercise book today, make a list of your achievements. You can use whatever has already happened during the course, for example:
- I went for a walk instead of watching TV.
- I wrote down my positive thoughts in the calendar today, making it another day in a row.
- Today I worked to be... (write something you are changing about yourself from the list created in the Chapter 7 exercise).

Expand your list of achievements every day.

Your Guide to Positive Life

9. MOTIVATION AS A LIFESTYLE

Motivation is a lifestyle based on your own rules regarding how you want to function. You alone decide how you want to live your life.

I'd like to share with you my proven ways to strengthen motivation:

Focus on your feelings
Imagine what you are going to feel when you achieve the goal. Happiness? Pride? Joy? Feel them right now!

Change the word „I must" to „I want"
For example, if you value cleanliness, you „want" to wash the dishes, because you like it – you will do it automatically, without effort. Using the word „must" can be discouraging by itself.

Make the goal attractive
You will never procrastinate on an attractive goal because you have too much motivation to work on it now! For example, if you associate ironing with your favourite music which sooner or later makes you dance around, you will find that you do not have to force yourself to perform this activity.

Focus on your values
Define what exactly is the tangible benefit of achieving your goal. What underlying values does it have? What will your life look like as a result? Feel it and you will see that work is the greatest motivator of all.

Describe your goal in your notebook according to my advice!

Your Guide to Positive Life

10. SELF-ESTEEM

Many people have a problem with self-esteem, which often results from lifelong experiences of hurt, disappointments and broken trust. **Today's tasks will aim straight for your heart.** First, you will find healing there and only then will you move on to build your sense of worth based on dignity and respect.

1. **Write a letter to your parents.**
   Our parents leave an indelible mark on our self-esteem. Thank them for everything they gave you. Although it can be difficult, in your letter write everything you would like to say to them, even if you do not have the opportunity anymore.

   If it helps, you can tear up the letter later and throw it away.

2. **Forgiveness.**
   Think about who you feel resentment for in your heart. Write that person's name in your exercise book and describe the situation that caused you the pain.

   Reach for forgiveness – it is absolutely necessary for you to move on.

   Think about what to do next with this relationship? Maybe it's time to give it up? You can make a one-month attempt to find out how that would make you feel. Or maybe it's time to have a sincere conversation to try and heal your relationship?

3. **The language of love.**
   When was the last time you told a loved one how you feel about them? Do the most important people know the place they occupy in your life? When was the last time you talked to them?

I know how difficult these exercises were. **You are really brave!**

Your Guide to Positive Life

11. WHAT IS EMPATHY?

Guided by empathy, we accept what is happening with the other person or ourselves without judgement or criticism. We simply recognize the emotion and acknowledge it: „Yes, I see you as you are!". We open our heart to myself and other people.

> „Empathy is fuel for intimacy."
> - Brené Brown

How to develop your empathy?
Focus on your immediate surroundings. Think about the neighbours that you meet every day and about the people you pass in the street. Remember! **We are one big family.** We have the same problems and the same desires.

Every time you meet a new person, think that they are a member of your family. Then the colour of their skin, clothing or beliefs will be irrelevant. **See them for who they really are.** Understand that on a certain level, we are all the same.

Furthermore, **begin to see all living beings as equal to you.** Although we differ enormously, we all have the gift of life and we have the same home – Earth.

It's time to open up to people you have so far subconsciously treated as strangers. **Your attitude will show others that they can do the same.** Thanks to this, the Earth will become more friendly to all of us.

Have empathy for yourself!
Focus on what you need – read, dance, write your own story. Be positive about life.

Celebrate small successes – write them down every day and at the end of the week, celebrate everything you have achieved!

Your Guide to Positive Life

12. FORGIVENESS

Once you know how important the empathetic attitude towards yourself and the world is, it is time to go back to forgiveness for a moment.

Return to your heart with new openness and remember:

*„God is love, God is truth.
When you judge God's creation, you judge the Creator."*

Write down in your exercise book the endings of the sentences below and finish the day with peace in your heart:

1. I forgive myself
   I forgive myself for thinking about my body...
   I forgive myself for thinking that my life is not...
   I forgive myself for thinking that my life is...
   I forgive myself for thinking that in my life I have never experienced...

2. I forgive my parents
   I forgive my mother/father that...
   I forgive myself for thinking about my mother/my father...
   I forgive myself that I did not appreciate my mum/my dad for...
   I fully understand and accept that my parents did what they thought was best for me. They expressed love for me as they could in the most beautiful way.

3. I forgive my loved ones
   I forgive my sister/brother/partner/friend...

Your Guide to Positive Life

13. EFFECTIVE MOTIVATIONAL TECHNIQUES

We are starting the last week of our work on the first path of *Your Guide to Positive Life.* Don't worry! I have already prepared more workbooks for you, in which step by step we will take an in-depth look at all the topics that I presented here.

I don't want you to lose your enthusiasm towards work. Your life is worth it!

I will show you my effective motivational techniques:
1. Set yourself small and achievable goals.
2. Plan with precision – do not doubt your real goal!
3. Always have a plan B – even though you work to the best of your abilities, certain factors will always be beyond your control. Plan B is your way to overcome them.
4. Always have a list of benefits that carrying out your plan will bring – it's an infallible source of motivation.
5. Visualize your success – you can use the 10 minutes method and take that amount of time every day to imagine yourself achieving your goal.
6. Be positive about everything you do.
7. Listen to motivating music, which will inspire you to act every morning.
8. Celebrate small successes – reward yourself for every small task done.

Check if your current goal meets all of the above points. If something is missing, this is the perfect time to add it.

Your Guide to Positive Life

14. STAYING IN TOUCH WITH YOURSELF

Congratulations! You have done a lot of work on your way to a happy and powerful life. If I were to leave you with one thought at the end of this Guide, it would be this: „Keep in touch with yourself." **Listen to what your mind, heart and body are saying. Respond to what they say!**

Go for a walk today, so that you can be alone for a while in nature. Think about it while walking, and when you return home, write down the answers to the following questions:

1. Who is important in my life?
2. Who makes my life better?
3. What do I like about myself?
4. What are my most pleasant memories?
5. What is my favourite book?

I often say: *„Many people can have my attention, but only someone special can steal my heart."*

Be someone special to yourself!

Repeat:
I'll get to it now. I have the best years of my life ahead of me.

Your Guide to Positive Life

15. DON'T WASTE YOUR ENERGY ON LOW SELF ESTEEM

The art of self-acceptance is largely about getting to know oneself. In order to be forgiving, you must understand why you think, feel, act, and behave as you do.

Not too long ago, you didn't even know yourself, so it was difficult for you to accept actions whose results you didn't see. You did not understand why you lacked motivation, why you were overcome by strong emotions and why it was difficult to make new acquaintances. Now you know yourself better.

Review your exercise book and calendar with notes from the last few weeks. You have achieved all of this by yourself.

Now it's time to stop wasting your energy on your internal critic, who may still want to inhibit your actions and take away your joy.

Think about the answers to the following questions and write them down in your notebook:
1. How will my life change when I become an optimistic, joyful and hopeful person? How will I feel when I achieve this goal?
2. How will my family life change when I change?
3. What things are the easiest for me to integrate into my life? Optimism, hope, joy? Why?

Carefully consider and finish these sentences:
1. I admit that I had difficulties with optimism/joyfulness in the past because....
2. I confess that I had difficulty in giving hope in the past because....

Your Guide to Positive Life

16. CARPE DIEM - ENJOY YOU LIFE!

This is the end of the exercises in the first volume of *The Guide to Positive Life*. I want to leave you with a few things, doing which may make your waiting for the second volume more pleasant. May it also be your reward for everything you have achieved in recent weeks.

1. **Detoxify yourself.**

    Drink a glass of water on empty stomach every morning. You can add a slice of lemon or a pinch of turmeric and a spoonful of honey. It's a great boost of energy!

2. **Find time to relax:**
    - get yourself a pleasant foot massage,
    - take a long, warm bath with relaxing music,
    - create your own relaxation area – surround it with your favourite colours and flowers.

3. **Plan your quiet time:**
    - maintain internal balance – remember about daily contemplation,
    - seek time to be in touch with yourself.

Please remember the morning and evening rituals.
Let it stay with you forever!

Sincerely,
Kasia Dorosz

Your Guide to Positive Life

Workbook 1

Your Guide to Positive Life